Journey to Dreamland

TIPS, TRICKS, AND FUN FACTS FOR A GOOD NIGHT'S REST FOR HAPPY CHILD

Carole C. Smith

Copyright©2023Carole Smith

TABLE OF CONTENTS

INTRODUCTION

Once upon a time, in a cozy little house nestled in a quiet neighborhood, lived a cheerful girl named Lila. Lila was known for her endless curiosity and boundless energy during the day. She loved exploring, playing with her toys, and going on exciting adventures with her friends. However, when the sun dipped below the horizon, Lila faced a challenge - bedtime.

Lila thought bedtime was boring. She believed that closing her eyes meant missing out on all the fun the world had to offer at night. Instead of going to bed, she would stay up late, playing with her stuffed animals, reading under her blanket with a flashlight, and building towering pillow forts.

As the days turned into nights and nights into days, Lila began to feel very tired. She couldn't focus on her favorite activities, and her friends noticed that she wasn't as cheerful as she used to be. Something needed to change.

One sunny morning, Lila's wise grandmother, Grandma Lily, came to visit. She had heard about Lila's sleep troubles and had a plan to help her understand the importance of sleep. She sat Lila down and began to share a magical story.

"Listen closely," Grandma Lily said. "I want to tell you about a wonderful place called Dreamland. In Dreamland, the stars shine like diamonds, and the moon sings sweet lullabies to everyone who closes their eyes. Children from all around the world visit Dreamland every night."

Lila's eyes grew wide with wonder as she listened to Grandma Lily's tale.

"In Dreamland," she continued, "there are adventures beyond your wildest dreams. You can fly with talking animals, visit candy castles, and have tea parties with friendly monsters. But there's one secret, Lila. You can only visit Dreamland if you close your eyes and go to sleep."

Lila started to realize that sleep wasn't about missing out on fun; it was about going on magical adventures in Dreamland!

That night, Lila climbed into her cozy bed, and instead of resisting sleep, she embraced it. She closed her eyes and imagined herself in Dreamland. She soared through the sky on the back of a friendly dragon, danced with firefly fairies, and even had a race with a super-speedy snail.

Each night, Lila looked forward to her adventures in Dreamland. She realized that sleep wasn't boring at all; it was a gateway to a world of endless wonder and fun.

With each night's adventure, Lila grew happier and more rested. She had more energy during the day to play with her friends and explore her world. And every morning, she couldn't wait to tell Grandma Lily all about her latest Dreamland adventure.

From that day forward, Lila learned to appreciate the magic of sleep. She realized that dreams were like secret treasures, waiting to be discovered every night. And so, in the little house in the quiet neighborhood, Lila became known as the girl who knew the secret to the most magical adventures of all—dreams in Dreamland.

And they all lived happily ever after, especially Lila, who now understood that the best adventures sometimes happen when you close your eyes and let sleep take you on a journey to Dreamland.

CHAPTER 1

Sleep

Sleep constitutes a crucial component of your daily routine, accounting for approximately one-third of your time. Quality slumber, obtained in the right amount at the appropriate times, is as indispensable for survival as nourishment and hydration. The absence of sleep hinders your ability to establish and sustain the neural pathways necessary for learning and memory formation, impeding concentration and rapid response.

Sleep serves a multifaceted role in various brain functions, encompassing the communication between nerve cells, or neurons. Remarkably, your brain and body remain exceptionally active during rest, with recent research suggesting that sleep functions as a form of housekeeping, purging accumulated brain toxins accrued during wakefulness.

While sleep is universally necessary, its precise biological purpose remains an enigma. Its influence extends across nearly every bodily system and tissue, affecting the brain, heart, lungs, metabolism, immune system, mood, and resistance to diseases. Scientific investigations reveal that chronic sleep deprivation or poor sleep quality escalates the risk of disorders such as high blood pressure, cardiovascular ailments, diabetes, depression, and obesity.

Sleep, an intricate and dynamic process, wields a profound impact on your overall functionality, a realm that scientists are progressively elucidating. This pamphlet elucidates the regulation of your sleep needs and unveils the intricate processes unfolding in the brain during slumber.

Approximately one-third of our lives is dedicated to slumber, an indispensable and involuntary process vital for our effective functioning. It stands as an elemental need on par with eating, drinking, and breathing, serving as a cornerstone of robust mental and physical well-being. Sleep not only rejuvenates our bodies but also facilitates the restoration and repair of our brains.

Within the realm of sleep, we engage in information processing, memory consolidation, and a gamut of maintenance procedures that prepare us for the rigors of the day. The significance of sleep reverberates not only in the health of individuals but also in the collective public health of the population.

Ensuring that we receive an appropriate amount of sleep, coupled with its quality, becomes a universal imperative. The ideal amount of sleep varies among individuals, contingent on their unique needs, driven by their personal sleepiness levels and sleep patterns. Sleepiness, in turn, is intricately linked to our innate drive for slumber, while our sleep pattern pertains to the rhythm and regularity of our sleep routines. Establishing a consistent sleep pattern enhances our ability to fall asleep at the same time each day.

Sleep, despite its ubiquity, remains a mystery in many facets to the scientific community. Throughout the sleep cycle, our bodies traverse various processes and stages. Optimal sleep quality results from a sufficient duration spent in all these stages, including the rejuvenating deep sleep phase.

Sustained poor sleep yields immediate recognizable consequences, encompassing fatigue, drowsiness, diminished concentration, memory lapses, and irritability.

A substantial segment of the population, up to one-third, grapples with insomnia—characterized by inadequate or poor-quality sleep. Insomnia can adversely impact mood, energy levels, concentration, relationships, and daytime functioning.

The nexus between sleep and health is profound; compromised sleep can amplify health risks, while poor health can hinder slumber. Common mental health ailments like anxiety and depression often underlie sleep problems. In such cases, addressing both the mental health issue and sleep disorder concurrently proves most effective. Deepening our comprehension of the sleep process is crucial to ensure consistent, high-quality sleep.

CHAPTER 2

Kids and sleep

Juliet's Sleepy Adventure

In a small town called Dream ville, there lived a girl named Juliet. Juliet was a curious and adventurous kid who loved exploring and discovering new things during the day. But when the sun went down, Juliet thought sleep was boring. She didn't want to close her eyes and miss out on all the exciting things that happened at night.

Instead of going to bed, Juliet would stay up late, playing with her toys, reading books under her blanket with a flashlight, and sometimes even building towering pillow forts.

As the days turned into nights and the nights into days, Juliet started feeling very tired. She couldn't concentrate on her favorite activities, and her friends noticed that she wasn't as cheerful as she used to be. Something needed to change.

One sunny morning, Juliet's wise grandma, Grandma Lullaby, came to visit. She had heard about Juliet's sleep troubles and had a plan to help her understand the importance of sleep. She sat Juliet down and began to share a magical story.

"Listen closely," Grandma Lullaby said. "I want to tell you about a fantastic place called Dreamland. In Dreamland, the stars sparkle like diamonds, and the moon sings sweet lullabies to everyone who closes their eyes. Children from all around the world visit Dreamland every night, Juliet."

Juliet's eyes grew wide with curiosity as she listened to Grandma Lullaby's tale.

"In Dreamland," she continued, "there are adventures beyond your wildest dreams. You can fly with talking animals, visit candy castles, and have tea parties with friendly monsters. But there's one secret, Juliet. You can only visit Dreamland if you close your eyes and go to sleep."

Juliet started to realize that sleep wasn't about missing out on fun; it was about going on magical adventures in Dreamland!

That night, Juliet climbed into her cozy bed, and instead of resisting sleep, she embraced it. She closed her eyes and imagined herself in Dreamland. She soared through the sky on the back of a friendly dragon, danced with firefly fairies, and even had a race with a super-speedy snail.

Each night, Juliet looked forward to her adventures in Dreamland. She realized that sleep wasn't boring at all; it was a gateway to a world of endless wonder and fun.

With each night's adventure, Juliet grew happier and more rested. She had more energy during the day to play with her friends and explore her world. And every morning, she couldn't wait to tell Grandma Lullaby all about her latest Dreamland adventure.

From that day forward, Juliet learned to appreciate the magic of sleep. She realized that dreams were like secret treasures, waiting to be discovered every night. And so, in the town of Dream ville, Juliet became known as the kid who knew the secret to the most magical adventures of all dreams in Dreamland.

And they all lived happily ever after, especially Juliet, who now understood that the best adventures sometimes happen when you close your eyes and let sleep take you on a journey to Dreamland.

The ABCs of Kids and Sleep

Good sleep habits start early and set the foundation for a lifetime of healthy sleep. Prioritizing your child's sleep is an investment in their well-being and happiness. If you are a parent, guardian, or caregiver wondering about the importance of sleep for kids? Let's dive into the world of kids and sleep, from A to Z.

A - Amount of Sleep

Kids need more sleep than adults. Depending on their age, children typically require 9-14 hours of sleep each night.

B - Bedtime Routine

Establishing a consistent bedtime routine helps signal to kids that it's time to wind down. Activities like reading a bedtime story or taking a warm bath can make bedtime more enjoyable.

C - Caffeine

Limit your child's caffeine intake, especially in the afternoon and evening, as it can interfere with sleep.

D - Dreamland Adventures

Sleep is when kids embark on exciting adventures in their dreams. Encourage them to share their dreams in the morning to spark creativity and imagination.

E - Electronics

Limit screen time before bedtime. The blue light emitted by phones, tablets, and computers can disrupt the body's natural sleep-wake cycle.

F - Fear of the Dark

Many kids experience a fear of the dark. Nightlights or a comforting stuffed animal can provide a sense of security.

G - Growth and Development

Sleep plays a crucial role in a child's health, growth, and development. The body releases growth hormones during deep sleep.

H - Healthy Sleep Environment

Ensure your child's sleep environment is comfortable. A cool, dark room with a comfortable mattress and pillows can promote better sleep.

I - Individual Needs

Every child is unique. Some may need more sleep than others. Pay attention to your child's cues and adjust their bedtime accordingly.

J - Just Right

Finding the right balance between too much and too little sleep is essential. Oversleeping can also lead to grogginess.

K - Knowledge

Teach kids about the importance of sleep. Explain how it helps their bodies and brains stay healthy and ready for the day ahead.

L - Lovey or Blanket

Many kids have a favorite lovey or blanket that provides comfort and security at bedtime.

M - Melatonin

Melatonin is a hormone that helps regulate sleep-wake cycles and routine. Consult with a healthcare provider before giving melatonin supplements to children.

N - Naps

Daytime naps can be helpful for younger kids, but make sure they're not too long or too close to bedtime, as they can interfere with nighttime sleep.

O - Observe Sleep Patterns

Keep an eye on your child's sleep patterns. If you notice persistent sleep problems, consult a pediatrician.

P - Patience

Establishing good sleep habits takes time and patience. Be consistent and supportive as you work on improving your child's sleep routine.

Q - Quality Over Quantity

Focus on the quality of sleep rather than just the number of hours. Restful sleep is key.

R - Regular Schedule:

Stick to a consistent sleep schedule. This helps regulate your child's internal clock.

S - Snoring

If your child snores regularly or loudly, it could be a sign of a sleep disorder. Consult a healthcare professional.

T - Technology-Free Zone
Make your child's bedroom a technology-free zone to minimize distractions.

U - Understanding Dreams
Help your child understand that dreams are a natural part of sleep and can be fun and creative.

V - Visual Aids

Use visual aids like charts or stickers to create a visual sleep routine that your child can follow.

W - Wind Down

Encourage calming activities in the hour leading up to bedtime, such as reading, coloring, or listening to soothing music.

X - X-tra Comfort

Offer extra comfort and reassurance if your child has nightmares or fears that wake them up at night.

Y - Youthful Energy

A good night's sleep ensures that kids wake up refreshed and full of energy for the day ahead.

Z - Zzz

The sound of peaceful, restful sleep is one of the most beautiful sounds in the world. Ensure your child gets enough "zzz's" for a happy and healthy life.

CHAPTER 3

What Happens During Sleep?

Sleep is a common concern for parents, and its impact on the household's well-being is evident to new parents. The quality of their baby's sleep can have a profound effect on everyone. Additionally, older children who do not get enough sleep can experience difficulties with attention, mood swings, behavioral issues, and learning challenges.

Sleep comprises two main types: non-REM (non-rapid eye movement) and REM (rapid eye movement) sleep. These two types of sleep together form a sleep cycle. Infants primarily spend more time in REM sleep, and their sleep cycles are shorter compared to adults. As children grow, the time spent in REM sleep decreases, and their sleep cycles become longer. By the time children start school, a complete sleep cycle lasts approximately 90 minutes, resembling that of an adult.

The initial stages of non-REM sleep, stages 1 and 2, are considered light sleep:

1. Easy awakenings are possible.

2. Eye movements slow down, and heart rate, as well as breathing, become slower. Body temperature also decreases.

Stage 3 of non-REM sleep is classified as deep sleep:

1. Awakening someone during this stage is more challenging, and upon waking, individuals often feel groggy and disoriented.

2. This stage is associated with night terrors, sleepwalking, and bed-wetting. It's also the most restorative stage of sleep, during which the body releases growth and development hormones.

In the final stage of the sleep cycle, REM sleep:

1. Rapid eye movements occur beneath closed eyelids, breathing becomes faster, and the heart

rate increases. Physical movements of the arms and legs are restricted during REM sleep.

2. This stage is when our most vivid dreams take place.

3. REM sleep plays a crucial role in memory consolidation and learning.

How Much Sleep Do Kids Need?

Depending on their age, children require different amounts of sleep. A child's general health and physical and mental development depend on getting enough sleep. According to research, kids who get enough sleep show improvements in attention, behavior, learning, memory, emotional regulation, mental health, Physical health, and overall quality of life.

General guidelines for the recommended amount of sleep by age:

Newborns (0-3 months): Newborns typically need 14-17 hours of sleep per day, but it's highly irregular and occurs in short periods because they wake up frequently to eat.

Infants (4-11 months): Infants require about 12-15 hours of sleep per day. As they get older, they usually begin to consolidate their sleep into longer periods at night.

Toddlers (1-2 years): Toddlers need about 11-14 hours of sleep per day. They usually start transitioning from two daytime naps to one longer afternoon nap during this stage.

Preschoolers (3-5 years): Preschool-aged children typically require 10-13 hours of sleep per night. Most children in this age group no longer need daytime naps, although some may still benefit from a short nap.

School-age children (6-12 years): School-age kids generally need 9-12 hours of sleep per night. It's important to establish a consistent sleep schedule to ensure they get enough rest as busy school routines can sometimes lead to insufficient sleep.

Teenagers (13-18 years): Teenagers need 8-10 hours of sleep per night, but many struggle to get enough due to academic, extracurricular, and social demands. Adolescents often experience a shift in their circadian rhythm, which can make it challenging for them to fall asleep early in the evening.

These guidelines and individual sleep needs can vary. Some children may need slightly more or less sleep than the average for their age group. To determine if a child is getting enough sleep, it's essential to consider their individual needs and pay attention to signs of sleep deprivation, such as irritability, difficulty concentrating, and excessive daytime sleepiness.

Establishing a consistent bedtime routine and creating a sleep-friendly environment (e.g., a dark, quiet, and comfortable bedroom) can help children develop healthy sleep habits. If you have concerns about your child's sleep patterns or if they consistently struggle with sleep-related issues, consider consulting a pediatrician or a sleep specialist for guidance and support.

Newborns lack a developed sense of day and night, leading them to sleep throughout the day and night. Due to their small stomachs, they frequently wake up to feed, regardless of the time.

Regarding the duration of a newborn's sleep, the National Sleep Foundation recommends that they should ideally get 14–17 hours of sleep within a 24-hour period. Some newborns may sleep as much as 18–19 hours a day.

These infants typically wake up every few hours for feeding. Breastfed babies tend to feed more frequently, typically every 2–3 hours, while bottle-fed babies might go about 3–4 hours between feeds.

It's important to note that newborns who sleep for extended periods should be gently roused for feeding. Until they demonstrate healthy weight gain, which usually occurs within the first couple of weeks, it's advisable to wake your baby every 3–4 hours for feedings. After this initial period, it becomes acceptable to allow your baby to sleep for longer stretches during the night.

The initial months of a baby's life can be particularly demanding for parents, often requiring them to attend to their infant multiple times during the night. It's essential to remember that each baby's sleep pattern is unique, and while some may start sleeping for longer periods (5–6 hours at a stretch) by 2–3 months of age, others might take longer to establish this pattern.

Safe Sleeping Practices for Babies

During the initial weeks of a baby's life, some parents opt for room-sharing, where the baby's crib, portable crib, play yard, or bassinet is placed in the parents' bedroom instead of a separate nursery. This proximity facilitates feeding, comforting, and nighttime monitoring. The American Academy of Pediatrics (AAP) recommends room-sharing without bed-sharing, as bed-sharing increases the risk of Sudden Infant Death Syndrome (SIDS) and other sleep-related dangers.

For a secure sleep environment for your baby, adhere to these guidelines:

1. Always place your baby on their back to sleep, avoiding the stomach or side positions. This practice has significantly reduced the rate of SIDS since the AAP's recommendation in 1992.
2. Use a firm, flat sleep surface and ensure the mattress has a snugly fitting sheet.
3. Avoid placing any other items in the crib or bassinet, including plush toys, pillows, blankets, loose sheets, quilts, comforters, sheepskins, and bumper pads.
4. Dress your baby appropriately for the room temperature and avoid over-bundling. Never cover your baby's head while they're sleeping, and be vigilant for signs of overheating, like sweating or feeling excessively warm.
5. Keep your baby away from secondhand smoke, it increases the risk of Sudden infant death syndrome (SIDS).

6. Offer a pacifier at sleep time, but don't force it. If it falls out during sleep, there's no need to replace it, especially if you're breastfeeding; wait until breastfeeding is well-established.

7. Eliminate potential hazards such as items with cords, ties, ribbons, or sharp edges that could pose risks in the crib.

8. Avoid letting your baby sleep in products not designed for sleeping, like car seats, boppy pillows, or infant loungers.

9. Do not use products or devices that claim to reduce the risk of SIDS, such as sleep positioners or monitors that track heart rate and breathing. None of these products have proven effectiveness.

10. Refrain from using weighted blankets, sleepers, or swaddles on or near your baby.

11. Ensure that all sleep surfaces and products meet federal safety standards and have been approved by the U.S. Consumer Product Safety Commission (CPSC).

Newborns naturally follow their own schedule, and over the coming weeks to months, you and your baby will establish a routine. It may take a while for your baby to distinguish between night and day. While there's no way to expedite this process, maintaining a calm and quiet atmosphere during nighttime feedings and diaper changes is beneficial. Dim the lights and avoid stimulating your baby with play or conversation to convey that nighttime is for sleeping. If possible, encourage your baby to fall asleep in the crib at night to associate it with sleep.

Resist the urge to keep your baby awake during the day in the hope of better nighttime sleep. Overly tired infants often experience more difficulty sleeping at night compared to those who have had adequate daytime rest.

If your newborn is fussy, it's perfectly acceptable to soothe them with rocking, cuddling, and singing. Swaddling, which involves wrapping the baby in a lightweight blanket, can also help calm a crying baby. If your baby begins attempting to roll over while swaddling, it's a sign to discontinue swaddling. In the early months of your baby's life, providing comfort and closeness is not spoiling but rather a source of reassurance. In fact, babies who receive affection and attention during the day tend to experience less colic and fussiness.

CHAPTER 4

Creating a Sleep-Friendly Environment for Kids: Where Dreams Begin

Effectively achieving a seamless and prompt process of getting a child to bed can frequently be seen as a noteworthy accomplishment. As many parents are well aware, children often exhibit a tendency to prolong the bedtime routine by expressing reluctance, complaining, and objecting. The classic refrain of 'But Mom, I don't want to go to bed!' becomes all too familiar.

Hence, if you find yourself grappling with the challenge of putting your child to bed without resorting to multiple countdowns, repeated trips to the bathroom, an abundance of extra embraces, and numerous requests for water, it may be an opportune moment to reassess your overarching approach to bedtime. A great starting point is to reevaluate your child's sleep surroundings. Both the physical ambiance and the emotional atmosphere you cultivate significantly impact their ability to relax their body and mind in preparation for the night.

Now, let's explore some key recommendations, ranging from enhancing their sleep environment to establishing an effective bedtime routine.

Embrace Serenity by Eliminating Clutter

Maintaining a clutter-free environment in your child's room is essential, although it can be quite a challenge with little ones around. Experts unanimously concur that clutter and disarray not only serve as constant reminders of unfinished tasks ("I didn't put away my toys!"), but they also stimulate the senses, making it more difficult for the body to transition into a relaxed state conducive to sleep. A tidy space, in contrast, exerts a soothing influence, facilitating your child's journey into a state of drowsiness. Encouraging your children to tidy up after their daytime play not only instills responsible habits regarding the care of their belongings but also ensures a serene, clutter-free sleep environment.

Mind the Temperature, Especially for the Littlest Sleepers

Dressing your child appropriately and regulating the room temperature can be a subject of concern for many parents with young children. Devoting attention to this aspect is worthwhile, as research has underscored the significant impact of room temperature on the quality of one's sleep. Experts recommend maintaining a comfortably cool room, typically around 65 degrees Fahrenheit, as studies reveal that our internal body temperature experiences subtle fluctuations throughout the day, dipping slightly during the nighttime hours. If the bedroom is excessively warm or chilly, it can disrupt the body's natural sleep cycle, leading to early awakenings or restlessness. Discover the art of fine-tuning your baby's room temperature for an optimal night's sleep.

Keep It Dark or Maintain Dim Light

It's true that most children prefer some degree of illumination in their bedroom at night. Many will settle for a nightlight, while others may insist on keeping overhead, hallway, or bedside lights illuminated. Although granting them extra light to alleviate their fears of the dark might seem tempting, excessive light can hinder the natural body rhythms that induce sleep. As night falls, the pineal gland in our brains releases melatonin, the sleep-regulating hormone. This process is a key reason why children should avoid exposure to electronic devices or television screens during the hour before bedtime. Not only does the content tend to be stimulating, but the screen's light can be particularly disruptive, inhibiting the release of melatonin. If your little one struggles with total darkness, consider using a sunrise light, which simulates both sunset and sunrise and can help regulate their circadian rhythm.

Craft a Soothing Bedtime Experience

Bedtime should be a tranquil and serene affair for children. Strive to create positive associations with bedtime, their bedrooms, and the act of sleeping itself. While it may be tempting to use bedtime as a consequence for misbehavior, this approach can lead children to develop negative associations with going to bed. After all, who wants to relax in a place that reminds them of the last time they got into trouble?

Incorporate calming and soothing activities into your child's bedtime routine. For instance, one family I worked with made a habit of reading and listening to CDs from Lori Lite's Stress-Free Kids series every night. In doing so, they prioritized relaxation and the creation of a calm environment as central features of their bedtime routine. Similarly, you can read relaxation exercises to your child; Inner Health Studio offers some beautiful (and free!) relaxation scripts that you can print and share with your little one during bedtime.

Establish a Robust Routine

"Babies and children thrive on predictability and routine. And it really can make a significant difference to sleep patterns." Even in the midst of life's chaos, especially with a new baby or young child, the establishment of routines can provide a sense of stability for everyone involved. A consistent bedtime schedule imparts boundaries and security to your child, helping them better understand their day, which in turn promotes their well-being.

Consider implementing a series of steps leading to bedtime, such as:

- ✓ Tidying up toys

- ✓ Changing into pajamas

- ✓ Brushing teeth

- ✓ Saying goodnight

- ✓ Sleep

Over time, simply commencing with the first step can induce sleepiness in your little ones.

If your child frequently wakes up during the night, it's crucial to determine the underlying reasons. As previously mentioned, children thrive on routines, and they often develop habits that can disrupt their sleep, such as waking up for a night feed even when they are old enough to sleep through the night. These behaviors persist because they are associated with comfort. While easier said than done, breaking these habits necessitates not rewarding undesirable behaviors. If waking up results in cuddles and attention, there's no incentive for them to remain asleep. Minimize interaction during nighttime awakenings so that your child no longer perceives waking up as an opportunity to engage in something enjoyable.

Morning Routines Are Important

Lastly, the way you begin your mornings is as important as how you conclude your evenings. Children who eagerly anticipate the coming day are more likely to sleep through the night without interruptions. I understand that summoning the energy early in the day can be challenging, particularly when you're busy, but reducing stress in the morning can significantly enhance the quality of everyone's day ahead.

Avoid Screens

Refrain from bringing your laptop or tablet to bed, and limit your cellphone usage. Wondering why? Studies have indicated that the emitted light from these devices hampers the production of vital melatonin in both infants and adults, which is crucial for facilitating sleep. This underscores the importance of maintaining dim lighting. It's a prudent practice to keep all electronic devices away when you're ready to sleep.

Decorations

It can be quite tempting when setting up a nursery. The allure of vibrant hues on the walls or captivating artwork is undeniable.

However, it's crucial not to overwhelm the room with excessive decor. Keep in mind that young babies, particularly those with more intense temperaments, can find bright colors and an abundance of pictures overly stimulating. Surprisingly, research has indicated that colors like red and orange can induce feelings of agitation and discomfort in individuals. Bright colors may prove overwhelming, and even hanging mobiles can serve as distractions that are a tad too much.

If possible, opt for more subdued and muted colors in the nursery. These soothing shades can help create a relaxed atmosphere for the baby

CHAPTER 5

Bedtime Routines for Kids and Teen

Quality sleep is crucial during childhood, yet research indicates that as many as 20 to 30% of babies encounter sleep difficulties. If you're a parent or caregiver of a young child who struggles with insomnia, you understand firsthand the frustration of witnessing your little one's bedtime challenges.

One of the most effective methods to establish healthy sleep patterns for your child is by implementing a bedtime routine. The encouraging news is that it often only takes a few nights of consistently following a bedtime routine to observe significant improvements in your child's sleep.

Bedtime routines consist of a consistent series of activities performed every night before sleep. Their purpose is to help your child unwind and relax, effectively preparing them for a restful night's sleep. These routines offer a sense of security to your child and teach them the valuable skill of falling asleep independently.

Research has shown that children who adhere to bedtime routines tend to experience a range of sleep-related benefits. They are more likely to go to bed earlier, fall asleep faster, enjoy longer sleep durations, and experience fewer night awakenings. Remarkably, these improvements in sleep quality can persist for years in children who established bedtime routines during their early years.

Beyond enhancing sleep, bedtime routines also impart self-care skills and lay the foundation for cognitive abilities such as working memory and attention. Additionally, they foster strong parent-child bonds and may contribute to improved mood, reduced stress levels, and better behavior.

In the long run, these advantages translate into better preparedness for school, improved academic performance, and enhanced social skills. Conversely, those who do not establish bedtime routines during childhood are more prone to sleep issues and an increased risk of being overweight during adolescence. Initiating a bedtime routine right from the start with your baby paves the way for maintaining healthy habits as your child grows.

Creating a Bedtime Routine for Children

A children's bedtime routine typically involves three or four activities, such as having a snack, brushing teeth, changing into pajamas, and reading a book. It's important to follow the same order each night for consistency. To enhance the routine's effectiveness, gradually transition the household into a wind-down mode by dimming lights and turning off screens before bedtime.

Common bedtime activities that have been proven to promote better sleep include:

1. Providing a nutritious snack or bottle/breastfeeding.

2. Bathing or changing diapers.

3. Brushing teeth and using the bathroom.

4. Reading a book together.

5. Singing a lullaby or sharing songs.

6. Offering a gentle massage, cuddling, and rocking.

7. Engaging in a conversation about their day.

The bedtime routine should conclude with a goodnight kiss and turning off the lights. It's essential to leave the room while your child is still drowsy but not yet asleep. This helps them learn to fall asleep independently, reducing any panic if they awaken during the night and find you absent. Lastly, establish a consistent bedtime that allows your child to achieve the recommended amount of sleep hours for their age.

There are certain activities that can hinder your child's sleep and potentially lead to unhealthy habits. While each child is unique, it may require some experimentation to determine the most effective bedtime routine for your family. Nevertheless, when creating your child's bedtime routine, consider adhering to the following guidelines:

Do:

1. **Consistency:** Establish a nightly bedtime routine with the same steps as often as possible. The involvement of both parents is important when feasible.

2. **Keep It Short:** A bedtime routine for most children should last around half an hour, slightly longer if it includes a bath. Avoid prolonging it, as this can delay bedtime, especially on busier days.

3. **Daytime Routine:** Implement a routine during the day, including setting clear limits, which can result in increased sleep duration for young children. Ensure they get exercise, sunlight, and outdoor time during the day to aid nighttime sleep.

4. **Listen to Your Child:** While you're ultimately in charge, consider your child's input. If a part of the bedtime routine isn't working, be open to their concerns and make necessary adjustments.

5. **Follow Sleep Hygiene Rules:** Maintain a dark, cool, and quiet bedroom environment to promote sleep. If your child is afraid of the dark, use a dim nightlight. Transition to quieter activities in the rest of the house after bedtime to avoid disrupting your child's sleep.

6. **Make Gradual Changes:** When modifying the bedtime routine, introduce one change at a time and consider postponing changes if other significant life events are happening. Shift bedtime gradually by 15-minute increments as your child's sleep needs change.

Don't

1. **Start When They're Already Sleepy:** Initiate the routine before your child becomes overtired, as

overtired children can become hyperactive or grumpy, making it harder for them to fall asleep.

2. **Allow Screens:** Avoid screen time close to bedtime due to the disruptive effects of blue light on sleep.

3. **Let Them Get Overly Active:** While children should have opportunities to burn off energy during the day, avoid letting them become overly active at night, as it can make them too wired to sleep.

4. **Offer Sugary Treats or Caffeine:** Keep evening snacks light and healthy. Caffeine should be avoided as it can keep kids awake. Beware of hidden caffeine sources in items like breakfast cereals, chocolate, and pudding. Remove the bottle before your baby falls asleep if they are bottle-feeding.

5. **Read Scary Stories:** Avoid scary or mentally and physically stimulating activities before bedtime.

6. **Permit Weekend Sleep-Ins:** While tempting, significant deviations from the usual wake-up time on weekends can disrupt the sleep schedule, leading to trouble falling asleep on weekdays.

Bedtime Tips for Different Age Groups

- **Toddlers:** Address separation anxiety with comfort objects like stuffed animals or blankets. Allow them to make some decisions, such as choosing pajamas or a bedtime story. Keep the routine enjoyable and calmly say goodnight when it's time for lights out.

- **School-age children:** Encourage them to take on more responsibility in the bedtime routine, such as brushing their teeth and tidying their bedroom.

- **Teens:** Give them more autonomy over their bedtime routine, but monitor weekend sleep patterns to avoid disrupting their weekday schedule.

As your child grows, be flexible in adapting the bedtime routine to suit their changing needs and independence levels.

Bedtime Routines for Toddler and Newborns

Perhaps you've strayed from your reliable baby sleep routine, or maybe your family's nighttime schedule has always been a bit unpredictable. Regardless of the situation, establishing a bedtime routine for your toddler can make the bedtime process smoother, reducing the nightly struggle.

Here's a comprehensive guide to help you begin, along with some excellent bedtime routine activities to prepare your little one for a peaceful night's sleep.

Establishing a bedtime routine for your child is a practice that can be beneficial from a very young age. In fact, many experts suggest initiating a nightly routine a few months into the first year when an infant starts to establish a more consistent bedtime schedule. This routine can help babies gradually relax and prepare for sleep.

If you haven't already implemented a bedtime routine for your toddler, now is an excellent moment to begin. Both you and your child will soon appreciate the comfort and predictability that arises from incorporating a few soothing habits to close out the day

Even if your toddler isn't particularly enthusiastic about the idea of bedtime, there's a strong likelihood that she will take pleasure in a nightly pre-bedtime routine. Having a structured set of activities satisfies her desire for predictability, making her feel safe and secure while also giving her a sense of control.

Equally important, you'll likely discover that a routine can make bedtime a less contentious affair with fewer protests. Engaging in calm, quiet activities encourages your toddler to relax rather than get wound up, setting the stage for a peaceful transition into sleep. Additionally, she's less likely to resist when she knows what to expect.

While a routine may not transform your toddler into a perfect sleeper, it has a good chance of providing everyone in your family with the rest they need. A consistent evening routine helps your toddler go to bed at the right time, which can significantly reduce issues like overtiredness, nighttime awakenings, or early morning risings

Creating the Ideal Bedtime Routine for Your Toddler

The most effective bedtime routine for your toddler is one tailored to your child and your family's needs. In general, a successful evening ritual should be calming, predictable, and of sufficient duration to allow your little one to transition from active to relaxed. Steps you might consider

1. **Consistent Timing:** Establish a consistent start and end time for your routine. A relaxing bedtime routine typically lasts between 30 and 45 minutes, with a maximum of 60 minutes. Starting early

ensures your child is ready for sleep at their usual bedtime.

2. **Dim Lighting:** Keep the lights dim throughout the routine, as low lighting helps signal the body that it's time to sleep.

3. **Screen-Free Zone:** Avoid screens like TV, phones, tablets, and laptops for at least two hours before bedtime. Screen time can disrupt your child's sleep, so make sure your nighttime routine is screen-free and keep electronic devices out of the toddler's room.

4. **Bath Time:** Start with a warm bath as it has a soothing effect, signaling that it's time to wind down.

5. **Pajama Time:** Changing into pajamas is a simple way to indicate that bedtime is approaching. Let your child choose their sleep outfit if they prefer.

6. **Bedtime Snack:** If your toddler typically needs a small snack before bed, offer one before brushing

their teeth. Opt for light snacks that include both protein and carbohydrates, like crackers with cheese or peanut butter on toast.

7. **Teeth Brushing:** Brushing teeth is essential for oral health and can encourage cooperation when done at the same time each night.

8. **Quiet Activity:** Engage in calming activities like reading books, singing quiet songs, or gentle movement. Keep the atmosphere calm and serene; this is not the time for active play.

9. **Special Goodnight Ritual:** Create a unique way to say goodnight, such as turning off the lights, using a white noise machine, or tucking in stuffed animals. Offer hugs, kisses, and a consistent phrase like "See you in the morning!" before leaving the room.

Tips for Establishing a Toddler Bedtime Routine:

- **Gradual Slowdown:** Start winding down after dinner to help your toddler ease into the bedtime routine without starting it at high energy.

- **Timing:** Initiate the routine early enough to avoid rushing your toddler to bed. If she's consistently restless or overtired, adjust the timing as needed.

- **Consistency:** Keep the bedtime routine consistent in terms of order and activities so your child knows what to expect.

- **Soothing Environment:** Maintain a soothing environment with dim lighting, minimal noise, and no screens.

- **Transitional Object:** A small blanket or stuffed animal can provide extra comfort. Incorporate saying goodnight to her favorite comfort object into the routine.

- **Sleep in Her Room:** Encourage your child to fall asleep in her own room, avoiding falling asleep in your bed or elsewhere in the house.

- **Anticipate Needs:** Check if your child needs anything like a glass of water or a nightlight before leaving the room. Make this a regular part of the routine, but avoid accommodating too many requests that may prolong bedtime.

- **Patience:** It may take time for your toddler to adjust to the new routine, so be patient and stick with it.

- **Shortened Routine for Naps:** Use similar cues as your bedtime routine for daytime naps to prepare your toddler for daytime sleep.

A Bedtime Routine Chart

Consider creating a visual chart outlining each step of the bedtime routine with pictures. This can help your child understand and engage in the process. You can use pre-made templates or let your child get creative and make their own chart with your assistance

Toddler Bedtime Routine

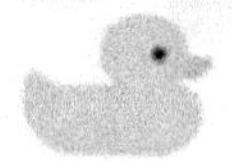

6:45 p.m.
Bathtime

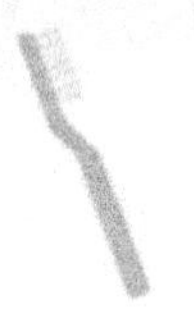

7 p.m.
PJs, bedtime snack, brush teeth

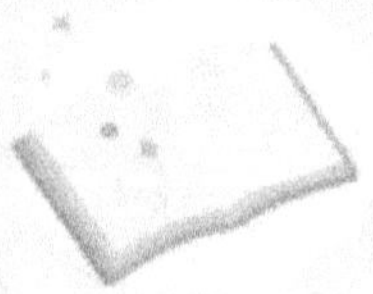

7:15 p.m.
Storytime, lullabies

7:30 p.m.
Lights out for bedtime

Establishing a bedtime routine for toddlers involves selecting a series of calming activities that prepare them for sleep. The key is to choose what works best for your family, with a focus on maintaining a tranquil, consistent atmosphere. Before you know it, your toddler will be guiding you through each step of the routine!

BEDTIME
Routine

- [ ] Brush your teeth and floss
- [ ] Tidy all toys
- [ ] Change into a comfortable sleepwear
- [ ] Set a sleep friendly environment
- [ ] keep it dark or Dim the light
- [ ] Turn off screens (Tv ipads phones)
- [ ] Read a book, Story time, lullaby
- [ ] Get into bed

CHAPTER 6

Nourishing Slumbers

How Food and Drink Can Promote Better Sleep for Children

In a world filled with screens, schedules, and ever-growing academic demands, ensuring that children get adequate and restorative sleep has become a crucial concern for parents and caregivers. Sleep is essential for a child's physical, emotional, and cognitive development. One often-overlooked aspect of promoting better sleep for children is their diet and hydration. The foods and drinks children consume can significantly impact the quality and duration of their sleep.

The Role of Nutrition in Sleep

Nutrition plays a fundamental role in supporting the sleep needs of children. Just as adults require a balanced diet for optimal health and rest, so too do growing bodies and developing brains. The right combination of nutrients can facilitate a smoother transition into slumber and ensure a deeper, more restful sleep.

Foods Rich in Tryptophan

Tryptophan is an amino acid that is often associated with promoting relaxation and sleepiness. It serves as a precursor to serotonin, a neurotransmitter that helps regulate mood and sleep-wake cycles. Foods rich in tryptophan can aid in the production of serotonin and, subsequently, melatonin, the hormone that regulates sleep.

Foods high in tryptophan include turkey, chicken, nuts, seeds, and dairy products. Incorporating these into a child's dinner can potentially help them feel drowsier and ready for bed.

Complex Carbohydrates

Complex carbohydrates like whole grains, brown rice, and oats have a mild sedative effect on the body. They help stabilize blood sugar levels and promote a gradual release of energy, which can prevent nighttime awakenings due to hunger or fluctuations in glucose levels.

A bedtime snack containing complex carbohydrates, such as a small bowl of oatmeal or whole-grain crackers, can help children maintain steady blood sugar levels throughout the night.

Magnesium-Rich Foods

Magnesium is a mineral known for its muscle-relaxing components. Incorporating magnesium-rich foods like leafy greens, nuts, seeds, and bananas into a child's diet can help relax their muscles and prepare them for sleep. Magnesium also regulates the body's stress response, reducing anxiety that might interfere with a good night's sleep.

Lean Proteins

Protein-rich foods like turkey, chicken, and tofu contain an amino acid called tryptophan. Tryptophan is a precursor to serotonin and melatonin, both of which play vital roles in regulating sleep. Including lean proteins in your child's dinner can promote a more restful night.

Calcium-Packed Foods

Calcium is essential for the production of melatonin, the hormone that controls sleep-wake cycles. Dairy products like milk and yogurt, as well as fortified plant-based options, can provide the necessary calcium for a good night's sleep.

Fiber-Filled Foods

Fiber aids digestion, and a comfortable stomach can contribute to better sleep. Incorporate fiber-rich foods like fruits, vegetables, and whole grains into your child's diet to prevent discomfort and indigestion at night.

Avoiding Stimulants

Caffeine and sugar can wreak havoc on a child's sleep patterns. Caffeine is a well-known stimulant found in coffee, tea, soda, and chocolate. Sugar, especially when consumed in excess, can lead to energy spikes and crashes, disrupting the sleep-wake cycle.

Limiting or eliminating these substances, particularly in the evening, can be highly beneficial for ensuring restful sleep.

Hydration and Sleep

While it's essential for children to stay hydrated throughout the day, managing their fluid intake in the hours leading up to bedtime is equally important. Avoiding excessive liquids right before bed can reduce the likelihood of nighttime awakenings for bathroom trips.

1. Timing Matters: Encourage children to drink most of their fluids earlier in the day. While it's important not to let them go to bed thirsty, reducing fluid intake in the hour or two before bedtime can minimize the chances of needing to wake up to urinate during the night.

2. Hydrate Smartly: Opt for hydrating choices that are low in sugar and caffeine-free. Water is the best option, but herbal teas like chamomile can

also be soothing and hydrating. Avoid sugary drinks and caffeinated beverages, as they can interfere with sleep.

Drinks for Dreamland

1. Warm Milk: The age-old remedy of warm milk before bed holds merit. Milk contains both tryptophan and calcium, making it an excellent choice for a soothing pre-sleep drink.

2. Herbal Teas: Herbal teas like chamomile and valerian root have natural calming properties. Steep a caffeine-free herbal tea for your child to help them unwind and relax before bedtime.

3. Tart Cherry Juice: Tart cherries are a natural source of melatonin. A small glass of tart cherry juice in the evening can aid in the production of this sleep-regulating hormone.

4. Water: Proper hydration is crucial, but avoid excessive water consumption right before bedtime to prevent nighttime bathroom trips. Encourage your

child to drink enough water throughout the day to stay adequately hydrated.

Foods and Drinks to Avoid

While certain foods and drinks can promote better sleep, others should be limited or avoided, especially in the evening.

1. Caffeine: Limit or eliminate caffeine-containing beverages and foods like soda, energy drinks, and chocolate, as they can interfere with sleep.
2. Sugary Snacks: High-sugar snacks and desserts can cause energy spikes and crashes, leading to disrupted sleep patterns.
3. Heavy, Spicy, or Greasy Foods: These can lead to indigestion and discomfort, making it challenging for your child to fall asleep peacefully.
4. Large Meals Before Bed: Eating large meals close to bedtime can lead to bloating and discomfort, making it difficult for your child to fall asleep comfortably.

CHAPTER 7

Creating a Sleep-Inducing Meal Plan

Putting together a sleep-inducing meal plan for children involves careful consideration of the timing, portion sizes, and specific food choices.

Here's a sample meal plan for an ideal day of sleep-promoting nutrition:

Breakfast:

- Whole-grain cereal with milk and a banana (providing complex carbs and magnesium)

- A glass of water or herbal tea

Lunch:

- Grilled chicken or tofu sandwich on whole-grain bread with lettuce and tomato (providing tryptophan)

- A side of mixed greens (providing magnesium)

- A glass of water

Afternoon Snack:

- Greek yogurt with a sprinkle of nuts and honey (providing tryptophan and magnesium)

- A glass of water

Dinner:

- Baked salmon or a vegetarian alternative (providing tryptophan and omega-3 fatty acids)

- Steamed broccoli and quinoa (providing magnesium and complex carbs)

- A glass of water or herbal tea

Bedtime Snack (if needed):

- A small bowl of oatmeal with a touch of honey (providing complex carbs)

Ensuring that children get a good night's sleep is vital for their physical and emotional well-being. Food and drink choices play a significant role in shaping their sleep patterns. By incorporating foods rich in tryptophan, complex carbohydrates, and magnesium into their diet and managing their fluid intake wisely, parents and caregivers can help children enjoy more restful and rejuvenating sleep. A well-balanced, sleep-inducing meal plan can be a powerful tool in promoting better sleep and overall health for children, setting them up for success in all aspects of their lives.

CHAPTER 8

Managing screen time

We can universally acknowledge the value of restful sleep, especially when tending to young children. Consequently, any activity that potentially disrupts this precious slumber deserves a cautious approach. However, a question arises: how many of us indulge in screen time before retiring for the night? This screen time might encompass watching TV, engaging with our smartphones or laptops, or even delving into an e-book on our e-readers.

The fundamental reality is that screens and sleep often prove to be an ill-fated combination, particularly for children who rely on sound sleep for their optimal growth and development. Recent research has indicated that, while certain amounts of screen time may not be as detrimental to mental health as once believed, disrupted sleep remains a persisting concern. In actuality, children frequently exceed recommended screen time durations.

Dear parents, it's important to acknowledge that if you've occasionally resorted to screen time as part of your child's bedtime routine, you are not alone. However, it's crucial to be informed about the complex relationship between screens and sleep in order to make the most informed decisions for your family's well-being.

Research findings emphasize that engaging in screen activities before bedtime, including watching TV, playing video games, or using phones and computers, can result in a reduction in the total hours of sleep and an increase in nighttime awakenings.

Screens may sometimes be necessary to ensure one child's safety and engagement while attending to another child's bedtime routine. Additionally, older children may require access to computers and mobile devices for completing homework assignments during the evening. However, it is important to also emphasize the importance of parental awareness regarding the influence of screens on sleep., "Consistently, studies reveal that screen time can lead to sleep issues in children of all age groups." according to a report in a 2021 systematic review on electronics and sleep, which highlights that evening screen time is linked to difficulties in falling asleep, reduced overall sleep duration, and daytime drowsiness, which is indicative of poor sleep quality

It's important to set limits on screen time for children and young people throughout the day to prevent a reduction in physical activity. While interactive games can be a way for children to socialize, it's crucial to also educate them about online safety. There have been increasing concerns about gaming and online addiction, and it's important to stay informed about these topics for the well-being of children and young individuals

Experts have also identified several ways in which screens may adversely affect children's sleep. One significant factor is the emission of blue light from screens. Blue light has the potential to hinder the production of melatonin, the hormone responsible for inducing sleepiness in our bodies. While blue light is beneficial for maintaining alertness during the daytime, its use at night, especially in devices like computers and televisions, can pose sleep-related challenges. Notably, blue light appears to have a more pronounced disruptive effect on the sleep patterns of younger children.

How does screen time affect toddlers' sleep specifically?

The content your child engages with on screens can vary in its impact, influenced by their individual personality. The lingering thoughts about what they viewed can keep them awake or even trigger nightmares that disrupt their sleep during the night.

Furthermore, screens might unintentionally reduce physical activity and encroach on time that could otherwise be devoted to fostering healthy sleep habits. As mentioned, screens have the potential to replace activities that are known to enhance sleep, such as maintaining a consistent bedtime routine, engaging in physical exercise, or spending time outdoors.

How to balance screen time

Balancing screen time has become a significant challenge for millennial parents, exacerbated by the pandemic and social distancing. Striking a balance between following health expert recommendations for screen time limits and the practical need for devices in daily life has been a source of stress.

Many parents find themselves in the middle ground, not wanting their children glued to screens all day but recognizing the utility of devices as parenting tools. The Family Link app, designed by Google, has proven to be a game-changer for many families. It empowers parents to stay connected to their children's online experiences by allowing them to set up a Google Account managed with Family Link, enabling parental controls on compatible Android and Chrome OS devices.

This app gives parents control, enabling them to manage content access and set time limits for screen usage. By effectively managing what and how much their children see daily, it helps reduce screen-time guilt while enhancing family fun.

Furthermore, Family Link allows parents to oversee everything remotely from their own iOS, Android, or Chrome OS devices, eliminating potential meltdowns when it's time to end screen time.

Screen time is an integral part of modern parenting, serving valuable purposes like expanding a child's horizons within the confines of home. The Google Teacher Approved apps program in the Google Play Store offers a solution by curating educational apps that are engaging and backed by experts.

Google takes these efforts a step further with Kids Space, a kids mode on select Android tablets designed to nurture children's creativity. It provides a library of expert-recommended, quality content tailored to a child's interests. This content covers a wide range of topics, from animals to cooking to cars, allowing kids to explore their curiosities while learning new things through books, videos, games, and apps. Parents can rest assured as these products are linked to their child's Google Account and managed with Family Link, ensuring supervision of device usage.

Exploring the Family Link app's parental controls from Google unveiled a crucial insight into crafting an effective screen time strategy for my family: Embrace the abundance of information available and ensure that our online time is genuinely enriching. This perspective resonates deeply with me as a practical approach to navigating the digital landscape.

Wind-down alternatives to screens

Electronic devices emit blue light, which can disrupt the body's natural sleep cycle and stimulate the mind. To prepare for sleep, it's recommended to avoid screens for at least 60 minutes before bedtime. Instead, activities like reading, listening to music, taking a bath, creative play, or enjoying audiobooks can help your child relax and get ready for sleep. "All kids wind down in different ways, so I would really recommend finding what works best for your child,"

Sleep hygiene encompasses the practices we follow around bedtime to prepare our bodies for sleep. These practices include:

Establishing a Regular Bedtime: Having a consistent bedtime helps regulate the body's internal clock.

Winding Down: Spend the hour before bedtime in relaxation and calming activities to promote a sense of calm.

Creating an Ideal Sleep Environment: Ensure the sleep space is comfortable with the right temperature, darkness, and free from disturbances.

Avoiding Stimulating Activities: Before sleep, avoid engaging in activities like vigorous exercise, heavy meals, or consuming caffeinated drinks.

Limiting Screen Time: Reduce screen time before bedtime to prevent the negative effects of blue light exposure.

For teenagers, keep an eye on their social media usage, as it seems to have the most substantial influence on their sleep patterns. it's also advised to avoid having screens in the bedroom. Research indicates that children who sleep near televisions or devices tend to get significantly less sleep. Furthermore, children who have both a device and a television in their bedroom tend to sleep even less.

CHAPTER 9

Coping with Nighttime Fears and Anxiety

Nighttime fears and anxiety are common experiences for many children. As the sun sets and darkness fills the room, a child's imagination can turn ordinary shadows into daunting monsters and unfamiliar sounds into sinister entities. These fears can be unsettling, affecting a child's sleep patterns, overall well-being, and even their daytime activities. As parents and caregivers, understanding and addressing nighttime fears and anxiety is crucial to ensure a child's emotional development and quality of life. This article will delve into the causes of nighttime fears, strategies to help children cope, and how to create a comforting sleep environment.

Understanding Nighttime Fears in Children

Nighttime fears and anxieties in children are a normal part of their development. Between the ages of 2 and 7, children often have vivid imaginations that can lead to misconceptions about the world around them. This fertile imagination, combined with a limited understanding of reality, can contribute to their fears.

Common sources of nighttime fears include:

1. **Darkness:** The absence of light can give rise to irrational fears in children. They may associate darkness with the unknown and believe that it harbors monsters or other scary creatures.

2. **Imaginary Monsters:** Children's imagination can conjure up frightening images of monsters or ghosts, which seem very real to them.

3. **Separation Anxiety:** The fear of being separated from parents or caregivers can intensify at night when children are alone in their bedrooms.

4. **Bad Dreams:** Nightmares are another significant source of nighttime anxiety. These vivid dreams can leave a child feeling distressed even after waking up.

5. **Traumatic Experiences:** If a child has experienced a traumatic event, their fears may manifest during nighttime hours when the mind is less distracted.

1. **Open Communication:** Encourage your child to talk about their fears. Create an open and non-judgmental environment where they feel comfortable sharing their thoughts and feelings.

2. **Validation:** Validate your child's feelings. Let them know that it's okay to feel scared and that their feelings are normal.

3. **Empowerment:** Help your child feel empowered by teaching them ways to cope with their fears. This could include deep breathing exercises, visualization techniques, or using a comfort object.

4. **Imagination Redirection:** Encourage your child to use their imagination in a positive way. Suggest

that they create a "protector" figure or a friendly character that can keep the monsters away.

5. **Bedtime Routine:** Establish a consistent and soothing bedtime routine for your child. This predictability can provide a sense of security and comfort for your child.

6. **Create a Safe Space:** Designate your child's bedroom as a safe space. You can use nightlights, soft toys, or a special blanket to create a comforting environment.

7. **Limit Exposure to Scary Content:** Be mindful of the media your child consumes, especially before bedtime. Avoid shows, movies, or books that may trigger their fears.

8. **Address Separation Anxiety:** If your child's fears are rooted in separation anxiety, consider gradual exposure. Start by spending a few minutes apart and gradually increase the time as they become more comfortable.

9. **Positive Reinforcement:** Praise your child for their efforts in coping with their fears. Positive reinforcement can boost their confidence and motivation.

10. **Professional Help:** If your child's nighttime fears are severe and persistent, consider seeking guidance from a child psychologist or counselor.

Creating a Comforting Sleep Environment

1. **Nightlight:** A soft nightlight can provide a gentle glow that dispels the darkness without being overly stimulating.

2. **Favorite Toys:** Allow your child to have their favorite stuffed animal or toy with them in bed. This can offer a sense of companionship and security.

3. **Calm Colors:** Choose calming colors for your child's bedroom décor. Soft blues, greens, and pastels can create a soothing atmosphere.

4. **Noises and Sounds:** White noise machines or soothing soundscapes can help drown out unsettling noises from outside.

5. **Comfortable Bedding:** Ensure your child's bed is comfortable and cozy. High-quality bedding can contribute to a more restful sleep.

6. **Bedtime Stories:** Read or tell your child a positive and lighthearted bedtime story. This can set a positive tone before sleep.

7. **Family Rituals:** Consider incorporating a family ritual such as sharing the best part of the day or a simple goodnight hug.

Nighttime fears and anxiety are a natural part of childhood, but they don't have to define a child's sleep experience. With open communication, understanding, and the implementation of coping strategies, parents and caregivers can help children overcome their fears and develop healthy sleep habits. By creating a comforting sleep environment and offering unwavering support, you can empower your child to face the night with confidence and tranquility. Remember that every child is unique, so finding the strategies that work best for your child may require patience and experimentation.

CHAPTER 10

Fun facts about sleep

Introducing fun facts about sleep can be a lighthearted and educational way to engage kids in learning about the importance of sleep.

Fun sleep facts tailored for kids

Sleeping Hours

Did you know that most kids between the ages of 6 and 12 need about 9-12 hours of sleep every night? That's like getting a full night's sleep and then some!

Sleep Cycles

Sleep isn't just one long, boring activity. It comes in cycles! Kids go through several sleep cycles each night, including deep sleep and dream-filled REM (Rapid Eye Movement) sleep.

Dreamland Adventures

During REM sleep, your brain is super busy. It's the time when you have exciting dreams and adventures. Sometimes, you might even meet your favorite cartoon characters or go on magical quests while you sleep!

Growing in Your Sleep

Sleep is when your body grows the most. So if you want to get taller, make sure you get enough sleep!

Cool Sleepy Brain

When you're asleep, your brain is actually cooler than when you're awake. It's like your brain takes a little break to cool off.

Blinking Lights

At night, your brain acts like a switchboard for blinking lights. These lights come from all over your body, like your eyes and your heart. They're like little stars twinkling while you sleep.

Sleepwalkers and Talking: Some people sleepwalk, which means they get up and walk around while they're asleep. Others talk in their sleep and say funny things. You might even do this, and it can be quite amusing!

Hibernation Like Animals: Animals like bears and hedgehogs hibernate during the winter, which is like a super long sleep. But don't worry, you don't need to hibernate like them. Your body is designed to get shorter bits of sleep each night.

The Sandman

You might have heard of the Sandman, a magical character who sprinkles sand or dust on your eyes to make you sleepy. It's a fun story, but the Sandman isn't real. Sleep comes naturally when you're tired!

Midnight Snacking

Eating a big meal right before bedtime isn't a great idea because your body needs time to digest. However, if you're still hungry, a small, healthy snack like a banana or a glass of warm milk can help you sleep better.

Dream Catchers

Some people believe that hanging a dream catcher in their room helps catch bad dreams and only lets good dreams through. It's a lovely decoration, even if it doesn't really catch dreams!

Sleepy Animals

Many animals sleep differently. For instance, dolphins sleep with one eye open, and birds often sleep while perched on a branch. It's fascinating how animals adapt their sleep to their lifestyles!

Technology's Impact

Did you know that screens like those on phones and tablets emit a type of light that can make it harder to fall asleep? That's why it's a good idea to put away screens at least an hour before bedtime.

Sleepovers and Giggles

Sleepovers with friends can be super fun, but sometimes you end up giggling and talking late into the night. That's okay once in a while, but remember, your body still needs its sleep!

Different Time Zones

When you travel to a different part of the world with a different time zone, it can mess up your sleep schedule. That's why jet lag happens, and it can make you feel a bit tired and confused until your body adjusts.

Synchronized Sleep

If you ever notice your pet cat or dog twitching or moving their paws while they sleep, don't worry, they're not having a bad dream. They're probably just dreaming about chasing a ball or running in the park.

Olympic Sleepers

Did you know that some athletes, like Olympic swimmers and runners, need even more sleep than regular folks? Their bodies need extra rest to help them perform their best.

Sleep Helps You Learn

Sleep is like a secret superhero that helps your brain. When you sleep, your brain sorts through all the things you learned during the day and organizes them so you can remember them better.

The Record for No Sleep

The longest recorded time someone stayed awake without sleep is about 11 days! That's like trying to watch a non-stop movie for over 250 hours.

Snoring Symphony

Sometimes, people snore when they sleep, and it can sound like a funny symphony. But did you know that even dogs and elephants can snore? It's a bit like their own lullaby.

Yawning Is Contagious: Have you ever noticed that when one person yawns, it can make others yawn too? Scientists aren't entirely sure why, but it's one of those sleepy mysteries!

Your Brain is Busy at Night: While your body rests, your brain is super busy cleaning itself up. It's like a magical cleaning crew that comes out at night to keep your brain in tip-top shape.

Babies Sleep a Lot

Newborn babies sleep around 16-17 hours a day! That's even more than grown-ups. They need all that sleep to grow and develop.

Dreams are Personal Movies

Dreams are like your own personal movies that your brain creates for you. Some people even dream in color, just like the movies you watch during the day.

Sleeping Upside Down

Bats are unique creatures because they sleep upside down. Hanging from their feet helps them stay safe from predators and ready to take flight quickly.

Noisy Dreams

Sometimes, when you're in a deep sleep, your brain can make your body move a little. That's when you might twitch, talk, or even walk in your sleep. It's like your dreams are so exciting, your body wants to join in!

Growing While Sleeping

While you're asleep, your body releases growth hormones that help you grow taller. So if you want to be as tall as a giraffe, make sure you get lots of sleep!

Sweet Dreams, Sweet Smells

Scientists have discovered that you can't smell things in your dreams. So even if you dream of the yummiest ice cream, you won't actually taste or smell it.

Moonlight Magic

Some people believe that a full moon can make it harder to sleep. They say it's because the moonlight is so bright that it tricks your body into thinking it's daytime.

Hugging Teddy Bears

Many kids love to hug their favorite teddy bear while they sleep. It's like having a little buddy to share your dreams with, and teddy bears are great listeners!

These fun facts about sleep can spark kids' curiosity and help them understand the importance of getting a good night's rest for their overall health and well-being.

Getting a good night's sleep is like recharging your superpowers. So, make sure you create a comfy, cozy sleep environment, and don't forget to thank your pillow and blankets for helping you have sweet dreams!

CHAPTER 11

Sleep in the Animal Kingdom

A Story

Once upon a moonlit night, in the heart of the sprawling Amazon rainforest, there existed a unique community of animals who shared an extraordinary bond through their love of sleep. This community, nestled deep within the lush foliage and whispering trees, consisted of creatures from all corners of the animal kingdom.

At the heart of the community was Leo, a wise old lion who had roamed the savannahs of Africa before finding his way to the Amazon. Leo was known for his majestic mane and his ability to snooze for hours beneath the gentle rustle of palm fronds. His favorite spot was a mossy clearing where the moonlight filtered through the leaves like scattered stardust.

Living next to Leo was Sammy, a curious sloth with perpetually drowsy eyes. Sammy was a master of napping, often hanging upside down from the branches, blending seamlessly into the forest's green tapestry. He was famous for his "slow naps," which could last an entire day.

In the canopy above, a family of fruit bats, led by Beatrice, thrived. They were nocturnal creatures who believed in the magic of dreams. Beatrice would regale her kin with tales of her nightly adventures in far-off lands, inspiring the bats to sleep the day away in anticipation of their own nighttime journeys.

Near the riverbank, Clara the crocodile held a special place in the community. While most thought of crocodiles as fierce predators, Clara was a gentle giant who cherished her dream-filled slumbers in the warm mud. Her snoring, heard for miles around, was considered a soothing lullaby by the other animals.

One day, a newcomer arrived—a chattering capuchin monkey named Max. Max was different; he believed in constant activity, day and night, and couldn't understand the others' love for sleep. "Why waste time sleeping when there's so much to do?" he wondered aloud.

Curious about this peculiar way of thinking, Leo, Sammy, Beatrice, and Clara invited Max to join them for a nightly slumber party. At first, Max was hesitant, but eventually, he gave in, swinging down from his treetop perch to join the others in the mossy clearing.

Under the gentle gaze of the moon, Max settled in, surrounded by his new friends. As the night unfolded, Max experienced something he had never felt before—an overwhelming sense of peace and unity. He listened to Leo's tales of African savannahs, Sammy's dreams of soaring through the canopy, Beatrice's journeys to distant lands, and Clara's comforting lullabies.

Slowly, Max drifted into a deep, restful slumber, and for the first time, he too became a part of the shared dreamscape of the animal kingdom. In his dreams, he climbed trees with Sammy, soared through the night sky with Beatrice, roared like a lion with Leo, and swam peacefully with Clara in the river.

When Max awoke at dawn, he felt rejuvenated, his heart brimming with gratitude for the newfound connection he had with his friends. He realized that sleep was not a waste of time but a way to explore the vast landscapes of the mind and bond with others in the most magical of ways.

From that day forward, Max embraced the beauty of sleep in the animal kingdom, and each night, the Amazon rainforest echoed with the harmonious chorus of snoring lions, slow-moving sloths, chattering bats, and a crocodile's soothing lullabies—a testament to the power of slumber to bring even the most unlikely of friends together.

BEDTIME ROUTINE CHECKLIST

BEDTIME
Routine

- ☐ Brush your teeth and floss

- ☐ Tidy all toys

- ☐ Change into a comfortable sleepwear

- ☐ Set a sleep friendly environment

- ☐ keep it dark or Dim the light

- ☐ Turn off screens (Tv ipads phones)

- ☐ Read a book, Story time, lullaby

- ☐ Get into bed

BEDTIME
Routine

- [ ] Brush your teeth and floss
- [ ] Tidy all toys
- [ ] Change into a comfortable sleepwear
- [ ] Set a sleep friendly environment
- [ ] keep it dark or Dim the light
- [ ] Turn off screens (Tv ipads phones)
- [ ] Read a book, Story time, lullaby
- [ ] Get into bed

BEDTIME
Routine

- ☐ Brush your teeth and floss
- ☐ Tidy all toys
- ☐ Change into a comfortable sleepwear
- ☐ Set a sleep friendly environment
- ☐ keep it dark or Dim the light
- ☐ Turn off screens (Tv ipads phones)
- ☐ Read a book, Story time, lullaby
- ☐ Get into bed

BEDTIME
Routine

- [ ] Brush your teeth and floss

- [ ] Tidy all toys

- [ ] Change into a comfortable sleepwear

- [ ] Set a sleep friendly environment

- [ ] keep it dark or Dim the light

- [ ] Turn off screens (Tv ipads phones)

- [ ] Read a book, Story time, lullaby

- [ ] Get into bed

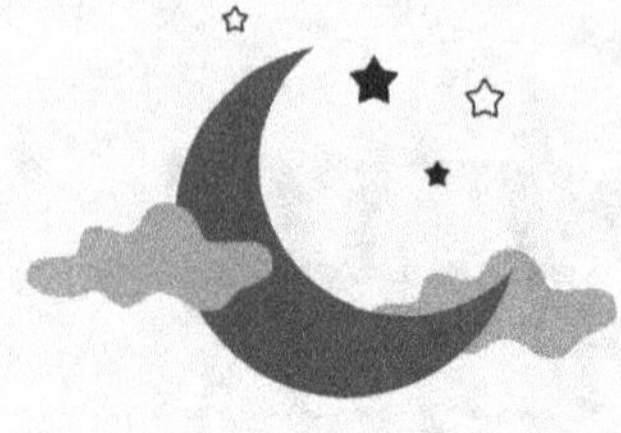

BEDTIME
Routine

- [ ] Brush your teeth and floss
- [ ] Tidy all toys
- [ ] Change into a comfortable sleepwear
- [ ] Set a sleep friendly environment
- [ ] keep it dark or Dim the light
- [ ] Turn off screens (Tv ipads phones)
- [ ] Read a book, Story time, lullaby
- [ ] Get into bed

BEDTIME
Routine

- [ ] Brush your teeth and floss

- [ ] Tidy all toys

- [ ] Change into a comfortable sleepwear

- [ ] Set a sleep friendly environment

- [ ] keep it dark or Dim the light

- [ ] Turn off screens (Tv ipads phones)

- [ ] Read a book, Story time, lullaby

- [ ] Get into bed

SWEET DREAMS AND

JOURNEY MERCIES TO

DREAMLAND.